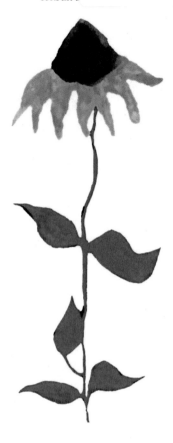

To my family and friends, thank you for sharing your world so generously and allowing
me to share mine. My life is blessed because of all of you!

YUIOPASDFGHJKLZXCVBNMQWERTOSDFGHJ
KLZXCVBNMQWERTYUIOPASDFGHJKLZXCVB
NMQWETYUIOPDFGHJKLZXCVBNMRTYUIOPA
SDFGKLZXCVBNMQWERTYUIOPASDFGHJBNM
QWERTYUIOPASDFG**H**JKLZXCVTYUIOPASDFG
HJKLZXCVBNMQWERFGHJKLZXCVBNMQWER
TYUIOPASDXCVBNMQWERTYUIOPASDFGHJK
LZBNMQWERTYUIOPASDFGHJKLZXCVUIOPAS
DFGHJKLZXCVBNMQWERTYFGHJKLZXCVBNM
QW**E**RTYUIOPASDVBNMQWERTYUIOPASDFGH
KLZXCQWERTYUIOPASDFGHJKLZXCVBNMT
HGJKLTEWLIOPASDFGHJKLZXCVBNMQWERT
YUIOPASDFADEUHJFNKOLNFHTIUYWMLHSG
UKBDSAZVOPHUIYEWQLMNBVCXZDRTYIOPH
CDRTYGTTUGFFE**R**DSHJLOBCRESGHJKLZXCV
BERTYUIOPASDFGHJKLZXCVBNMQWERTYUI
OPASDFGHJKLZXCVBNMQWERTYUIOPASDF
GHJKLZXCVKBNMQWYUIOPASDFGHJKLZXC
QWERTYUIOPASDFGHJKLZXCV**B**NMTHGJKLTE
WLIOPASDFGHJKLZXCVBNMQWERTYUIOPAS
DFADEUHJFNKOLNFHTIUYWMLHSGUKBDSAZ
VOPHUIYEWQLMNBVCXZDRTYIOPHCDRTYGT
TUGFFERDSHJLOBCRESGHJKLZXCVBERTYUI
OPA**S**DFGHJKLZXCVBNMQWERTYUIOPASDF
GHJKLZXCVBNMQWERTYUIOPASDFGHJKLZ
XCVKBNMQWERTYUIOPASDFGHJKLZMQWE
MQWERTYUIOPASDFGHJKLZXCVKBNMQWE
RTYUIOPASDFGHJKLZRTYUIOPASDFGHJKL
ZXCVKBNMQWERTYUIOPASDFGHJKLZXCVB

YUIOPASDFGHJKLZXCVBNMQ**W**ERTOSDFGHJ
KLZXCVBNMQWERTYUIOPASDFGHJKLZXCVB
NMQWETYUIOPDFGHJKLZXCVBNMRTYUIOPA
SDFGKLZXCVBNMQWERTYUIOPASDFGHJBNM
QWERTYUIOPASDFGHJKLZXCVTYUIOPASDFG
HJKLZXCVBNMQWERFGHJKLZXCVBNMQWER
TYUI**O**PASDXCVBNMQWERTYUIOPASDFGHJK
LZBNMQWERTYUIOPASDFGHJKLZXCVUIOPAS
DFGHJKLZXCVBNMQWERTYFGHJKLZXCVBNM
QWERTYUIOPASDVBNMQWERTYUIOPASDFGH
KLZXCQWERTYUIOPASDFGHJKLZXCVBNMT
HGJKLTEWLIOPASDFGHJKLZXCVBNMQWERT
YUIOPASDFADEUHJFNKOLNFHTIUYWMLHSG
UKBDSAZVOPHUIYEWQLMNBVCXZDRTYIOPH
CD**R**TYGTTUGFFERDSHJLOBCRESGHJKLZXCV
BERTYUIOPASDFGHJKLZXCVBNMQWERTYUI
DPASDFGHJKLZXCVBNMQWERTYUIOPASDF
GHJKLZXCVKBNMQWYUIOPASDFGHJKLZXC
QWERTYUIOPASDFGHJKLZXCVBNMTHGJKLTE
WLIOPASDFGHJKLZXCVBNMQWERTYUIOPAS
DFADEUHJFNKOLNFHTIUYWMLHSGUKBDSAZ
VOPHUIYEWQLMNBVCXZDRTYIOPHCDRTYGT
TUGFFERDSHJLOBCRESGHJKLZXCVBERTYUI
DPASDFGHJKLZXCVBNMQWERTYUIOPASDF
GHJKLZXCVBNMQWERTYUIOPASDFGHJ**K**LZ
XCVKBNMQWERTYUIOPASDFGHJKLZMQWE
MQWERTYUIOPASDFGHJKLZXCVKBNMQWE
RTYUIOPASDFGHJKLZRTYUIOPASDFGHJKL
ZXCVKBNMQWERTYUIOPASDFGHJKLZXCVB

HERBS.

An ABC Rhyme Picture and Book

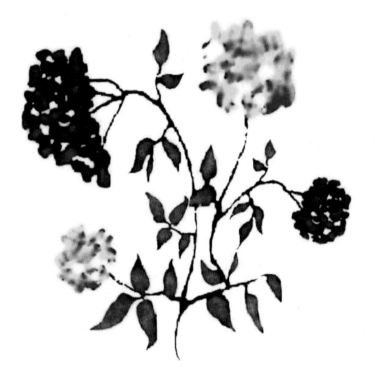

Tamara Gondre Lawrence, ND

For Malachi

I'm glad the sky is painted blue,
And the earth is painted green,
With such a lot of nice fresh air
All sandwiched in between.
-Anonymous

Now listen closely,
These pages confide
Certain truths about herbs
Verses written in rhyme.

Common and *Latin* names

Given below
Each herbal picture,
Just so you know.

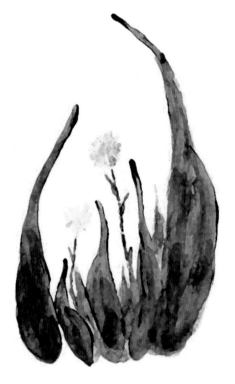

Aloe Vera - *Aloe barbadensis*

A is for Aloe.

Your friends you must tell,
Soothes burns on the spot,
Apply quickly the gel.

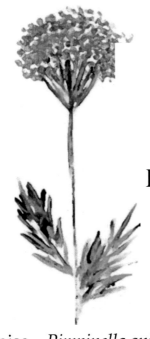

A is for Anise.

A taste sure to savor,
Eat or brew tea
For that licorice flavor.

Anise – *Pimpinella anisum*

A is for Arnica.

Be careful don't eat.
Collect flowers when hiking
And rub on sore knees.

Wolfbane - *Arnica montana*

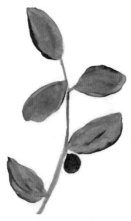

A is for
Ashwaganda.
It makes a calming tonic,
Combine with like herbs
For an action harmonic.

Ashwaganda – *Withania somnifera*

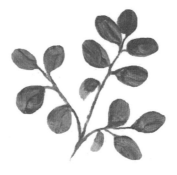

Astragalus – *Astragalus membranaceus*

A is for Astragalus.
Study well and retain
For its action, can help
Restore health or maintain.

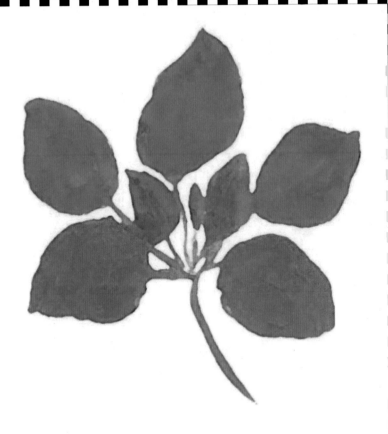

Basil – *Ocimum basilicum*

B is for Basil.

A wonderful herb,
In pizza or sauces
Adds a flavor superb.

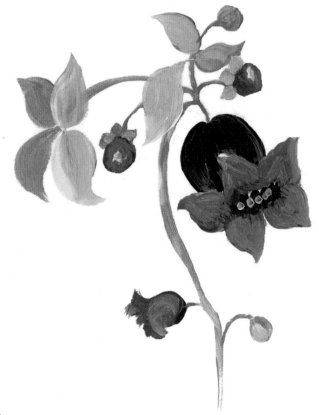

Deadly Nightshade - *Atropa belladonna*

B is for Belladonna.

This bell of the ball,
Will dilate your eyes,
So be cautious or fall.

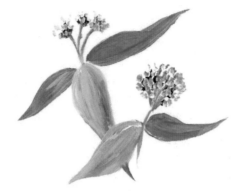

Boneset – *Eupatorium perfoliatum*

B is for Boneset.

Long tradition of use
To help feverish states,
Colds and body aches too!

B is for Borage.

Oil made from the seeds,
And its lovely star flowers,
Attracts plenty of bees.

Borage – *Borago officinalis*

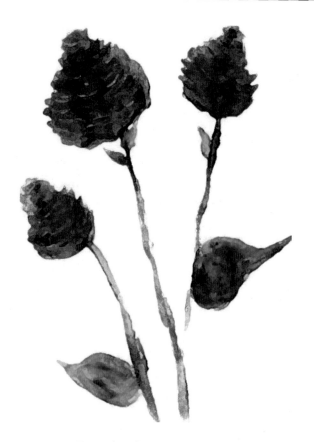

Burdock - *Arctium lappa*

B is for Burdock.

Best not to forgo,
The roots are quite hearty
And helps your skin glow.

C is for Catnip.
Or Catmint you'll find,
Not only for felines
But to quiet your mind.

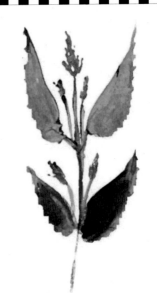

Catnip – *Nepeta cataria*

C is for Cayenne.
It may take a while,
But occasional use,
Turns a frown to a smile.

Cayenne – *Capsicum frutescens*

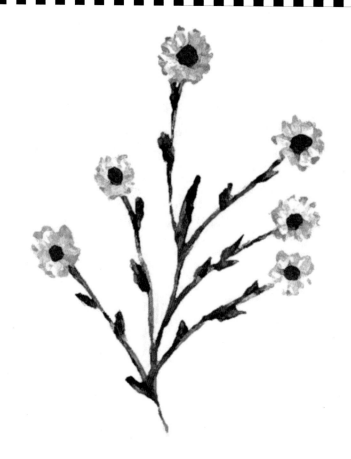

German Chamomile - *Matricaria recutita*

C is for Chamomile.

A quite popular tea,
Calms stomach and mind,
It's worth drinking indeed.

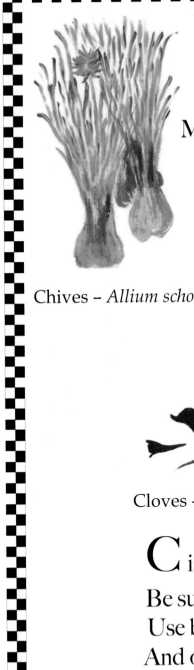

C is for Chives.

Many great chefs would say
A very fine herb,
Rich in vitamin A.

Chives – *Allium schoenoprasum*

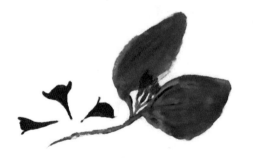

Cloves – *Syzygium aromaticum*

C is for Cloves.

Be sure to store some
Use buds to spice tea
And oil for sore gums.

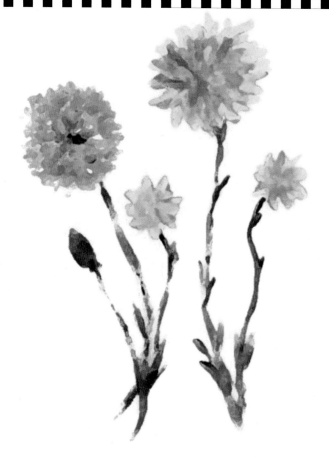

Dandelion – *Taraxacum officinale*

D is for Dandelion.

Remember this ballad,
Roast roots for herb coffee,
Mix leaves in your salad.

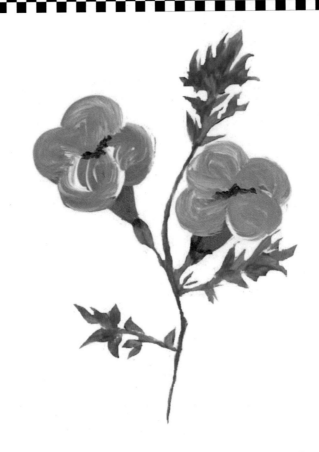

Devil's claw – *Harpagophytum procumbens*

D is for Devil's claw.

The berries can harm,
But the root eases pain
And spasms it calms.

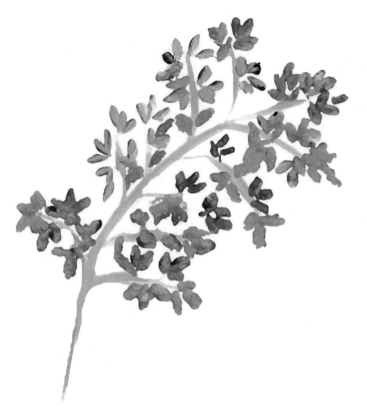

Dill – *Anethum graveolens*

D is for Dill.

Best when it's fresh
In soups or with pickles
Mixed with lemon juice or zest.

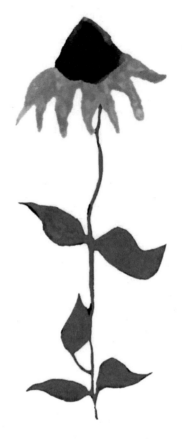

Coneflower – *Echinacea purpurea*

E is for Echinacea.

It might tingle your tongue,
But gives vigor when sick,
For the old and the young.

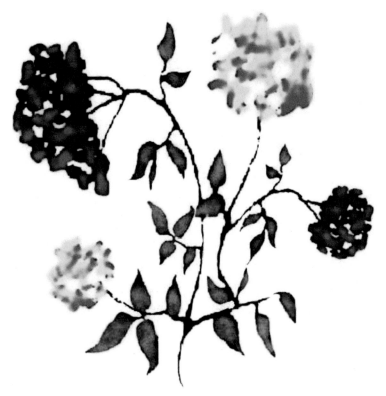

Elder – *Sambucus nigra*

E is for Elder.

An herb tried and true,
The flowers promote sweating
And the berries fight the flu.

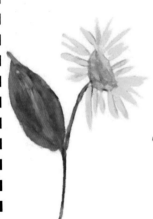

E is for

Elecampane.
It favors the lungs,
Though the smell of the tea
Is off-putting to some.

Elecampane – *Inula helenium*

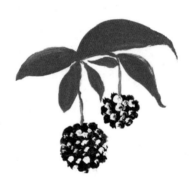

Siberian ginseng – *Eleutherococcus senticosus*

E is for Eleuthrococcus.
Say Eleuthro for short
Helps you adapt
To stress of most sorts.

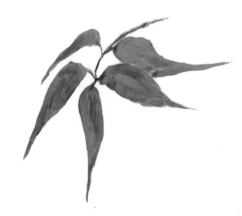

Eucalyptus – *Eucalyptus globus*

E is for Eucalyptus.
Essential oil is cooling.
Just relax and breathe in
Its fumes ever soothing.

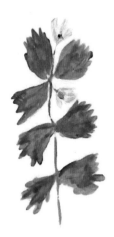

E is for Eyebright.
So, here's a surprise...
Eases eye inflammation
But won't brighten your eyes.

Eyebright – *Euphrasia officinalis*

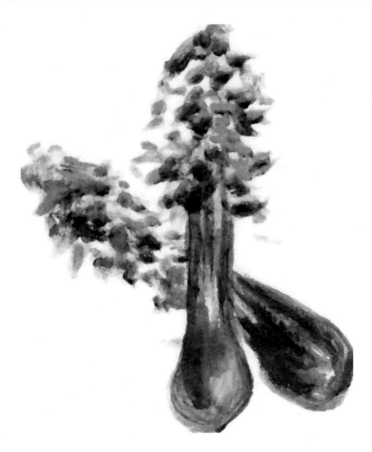

Fennel – *Foeniculum vulgare*

F is for Fennel.

Just chew on the seeds,
To freshen your breath
Or for gas pain relief.

F is for Fenugreek.
Advice you should heed,
When cooking soak first,
To soften its seed.

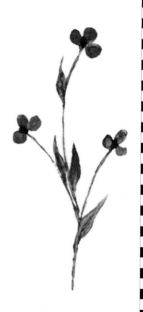

Fenugreek – *Trigonella foenum-graecum*

F is for Figs.
This fruit for the soul,
Will help you stay regular
Try the spread or eat whole.

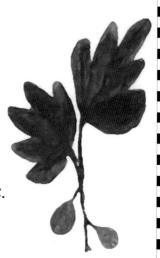

Figs – *Ficus carica*

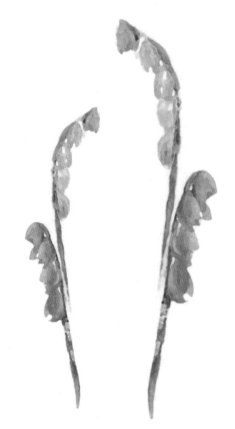

Foxglove – *Digitalis purpurea*

F is for Foxglove.

Its main claim to fame
Helps the ailing heart,
So, the experts proclaim.

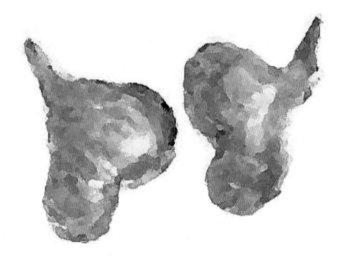

Garlic – *Allium sativum*

G is for Garlic.

Keep handy this gem,
It's usually stale
When out shoots a green stem.

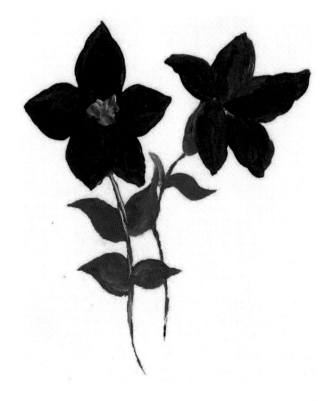

Gentian – *Gentiana lutea*

G is for Gentian.

An herb highly bitter,
For digestion just add
One drop per cup water.

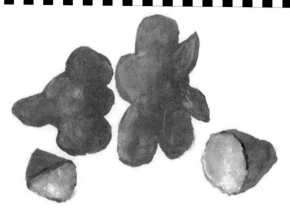

Ginger – *Zingiber officinale*

G is for Ginger.
There's no need to fret!
To calm a queasy stomach,
On this herb you can bet.

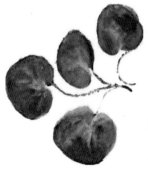

G is for Gotu Kola.
A low creeping green,
Cooks up just like spinach,
Just add butter and cream.

Gotu Kola – *Centella asiatica*

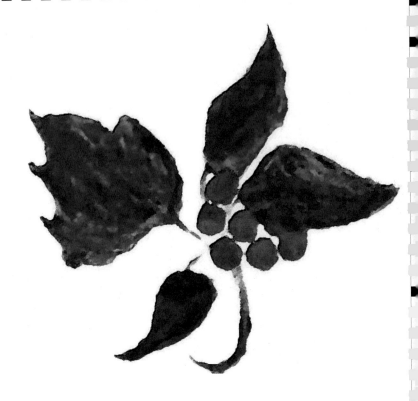

Hawthorn – *Crataegus species*

H is for Hawthorn.

A tree to preserve,
Pick berries for your heart
And the love you deserve.

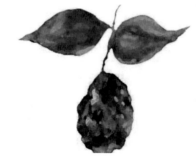

Hops – *Humulus lupulus*

H is for Hops.

Sleepless nights it may just quell.
The brew is a beverage
That many know well.

H is for
Horehound.

It's considered quite weedy
But for hoarseness you'll find
Great relief fast and easy.

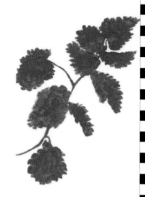

Horehound – *Marrubium vulgare*

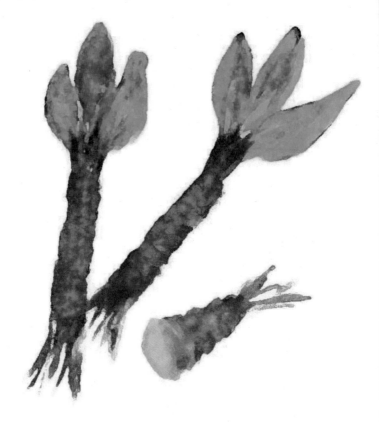

Horseradish – *Armoracia rusticana*

H is for Horseradish.

A good food to eat,
With a strong enough flavor
To give sinus relief.

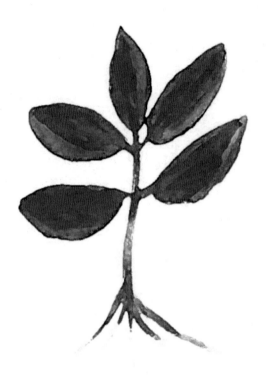

Ipecac – *Cephaelis ipecacuanha*

I is for Ipecac.

Minute doses excite
The stomach juices to flow,
And increases appetite.

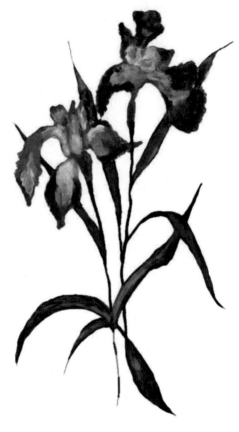

Blue Flag – *Iris versicolor*

I is for Iris.

Mother Nature adorned
With spectacular beauty
Yet a flavor most scorned!

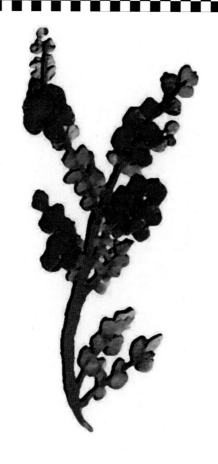

Juniper – *Juniperus communis*

J is for Juniper.

Their deep violet berries
Can flavor dark meats
And your favorite root veggies.

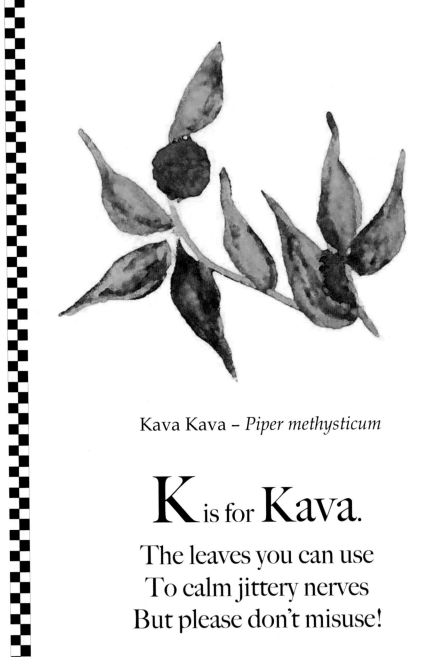

Kava Kava – *Piper methysticum*

K is for Kava.

The leaves you can use
To calm jittery nerves
But please don't misuse!

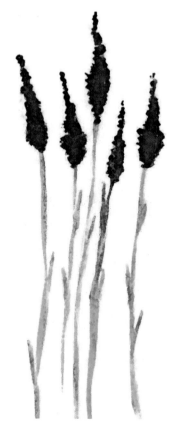

English Lavender – *Lavandula angustifolia*

L is for Lavender.

An herbal elite
That is useful for burns,
Apply quickly and neat.

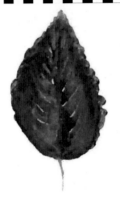

Lemon Balm – *Melissa officinalis*

L is for Lemon Balm.

It's true to its name,
The leaves smell of lemons,
And it calms nerves and pain.

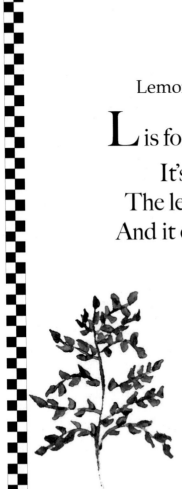

L is for Licorice.

It will sweeten your tooth,
But it's the ill and the worn
You'll find it behooves.

Licorice – *Glycyrrhiza glabra*

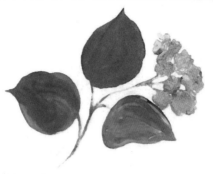

Linden – *Tilia tomentosa*

L is for Linden.

Its pale-yellow flower
When mixed with Chamomile
Gives enhanced flower power.

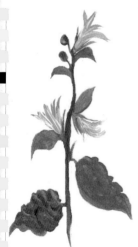

L is for Lobelia.

Use small doses for cough.
Slight nausea means
You've had more than enough.

Indian tobacco – *Lobelia inflata*

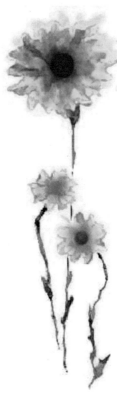

Marigold – *Calendula officinalis*

M is for Marigold.

You must practice your Latin,
Calendula, most say
For burns, cuts, and scratches.

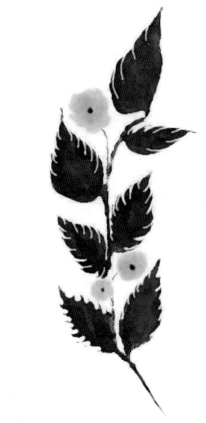

Marshmallow - *Althaea officinalis*

M is for Marshmallow.

The root soothes and cools,
Not the white fluffy stuff,
But like Slippery Elm gruel.

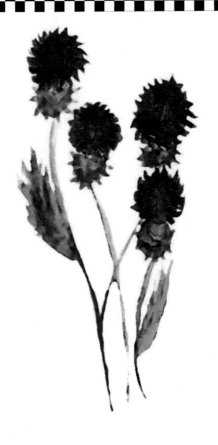

Milk Thistle – *Silybum marianum*

M is for Milk Thistle.

Seeds help to protect
From exposure to toxins,
Without harmful effects.

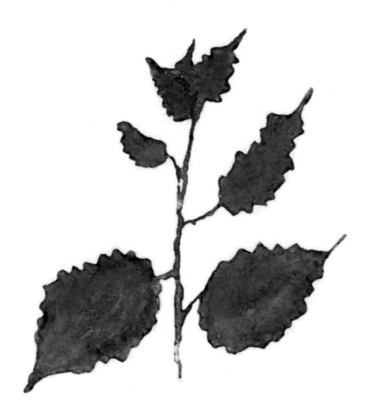

Stinging Nettles – *Urtica dioica*

N is for Nettles.

Simply handle with care,
The fresh leaves can sting
But it's food, so please share.

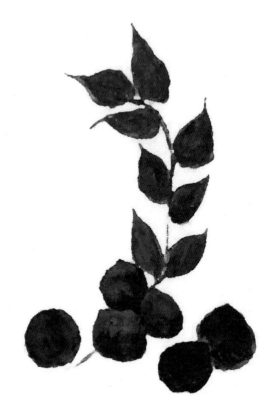

Nutmeg – *Myristica fragrans*

N is for Nutmeg.

It's best to buy whole,
Grind in milk before bed
If soon to sleep is the goal.

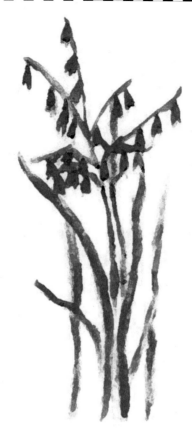

Oatstraw - *Avena sativa*

O is for Oats.

A great breakfast food
And for itchy dry skin
Or for lifting your mood.

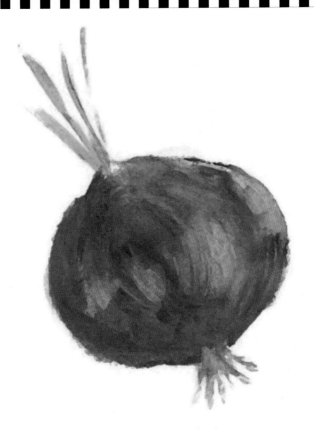

Onion - *Allium cepa*

O is for Onion.

A neat trick worth trying,
Freeze for 10 minutes
To keep you from crying.

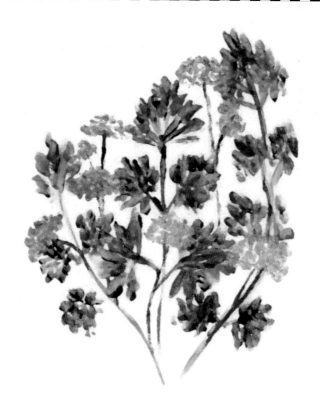

Parsley – *Petroselinum crispum*

P is for Parsley.

To find is a cinch,
But for Vitamin C
You'll need more than a pinch.

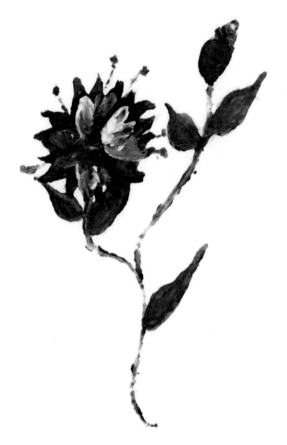

Passion Flower- *Passiflora incarnata*

P is for Passion Flower.

Do you need to unwind?
But this beautiful flower
Will help quiet the mind.

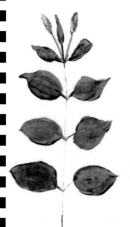

P is for
Peppermint.
It's easy to spot,
For the pepper and mint flavor,
Overshadows the lot.

Peppermint – *Mentha piperita*

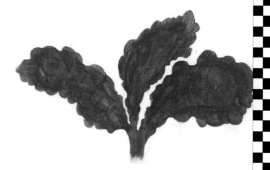

Kutki – *Picrorhiza kurroa*

P is for Picrorhiza.
Like Milk thistle you see,
Protects liver from toxins
Though prevention is key.

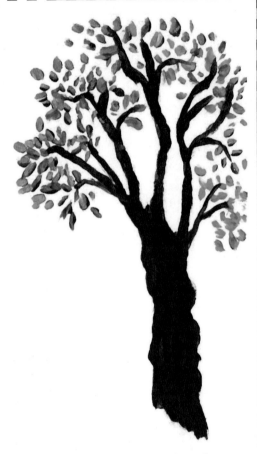

Quebracho – *Aspidosperma quebracho*

Q is for Quebracho.

It must be preserved
For the health of the planet
And future of herbs.

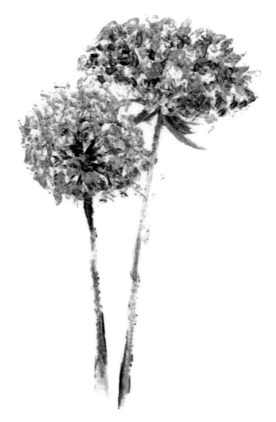

Wild Carrot – *Daucus carota*

Q is for Queen Anne's lace.

Be informed, not deceived
Resembles the Hemlock
That poisoned Socrates!

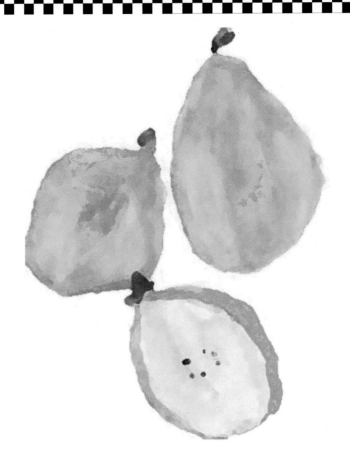

Quince - *Cydonia oblongata*

Q is for Quince.

A fruit worth a mention,
Whether roasted or preserved,
It's sure to sharpen your senses.

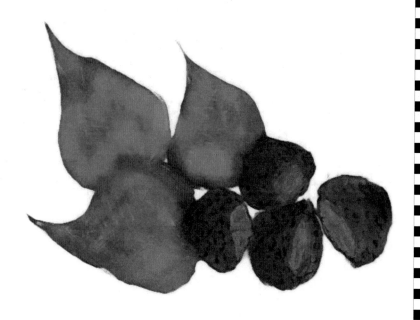

Red Raspberry – *Rubus idaeus*

R is for Raspberry.

Leaves relaxes smooth muscles,
And a handful of berries
Will help hustle your bustle.

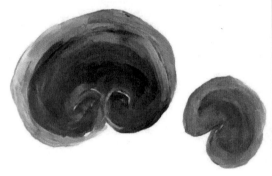

Reishi – *Ganoderma lucidum*

R is for Reishi.

A mushroom that grows
On trees and it will boost
Your immunity, if disposed.

R is for Roselle.

Caribbean custom will tell,
Steep the sepals and spice,
For the drink called Sorrel.

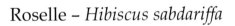

Roselle – *Hibiscus sabdariffa*

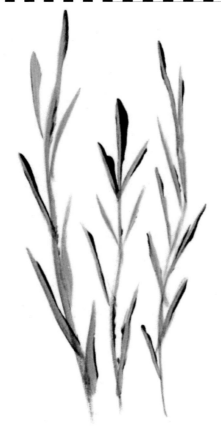

Rosemary - *Rosemarinus officinalis*

R is for Rosemary.

The name means remembrance,
Make a strong cup of tea
For drinking or hair rinse.

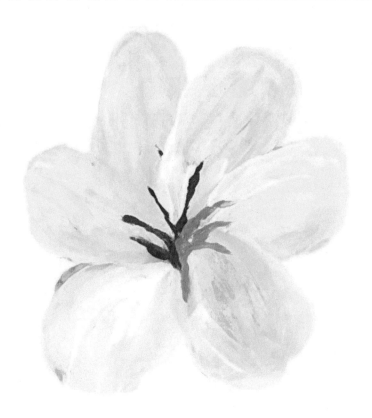

Saffron – *Crocus sativus*

S is for Saffron.

An elegant spice,
A few stigmas, though bitter,
Adds a fragrance quite nice.

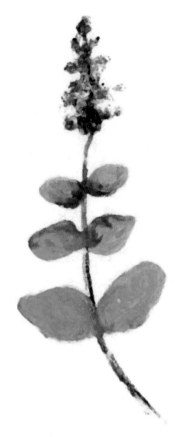

Sage – *Salvia officinalis*

S is for Sage.

The best of its kind,
Pray drink and eat
This herb for the wise!

Sassafras – *Sassafras albidum*

S is for Sassafras.

A fact you might hear,
Once a popular flavor
As the original root beer.

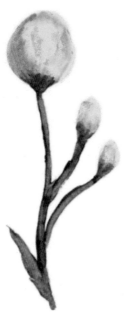

S is for Senna.

Shines bright as the sun,
But a few sips of the tea
Sure, to give you the runs.

Senna – *Cassia senna*

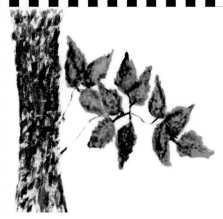

Slippery Elm - *Ulmus rubra*

S is for Slippery Elm.

Bark makes a rich gruel,
Add to porridge or pudding
For a healthier food.

S is for Sweet Annie.

A sweet smelling herb,
Use aerial parts
To treat parasites and worms.

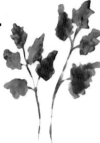

Wormwood – *Artemisia annua*

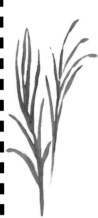

T is for Tarragon.

Chop through once, sharp and
clean,
So, the delicate leaves
Won't turn black but stay green.

Tarragon - *Artemisia dracunuclus*

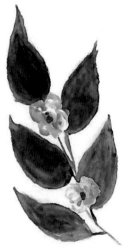

T is for Tea.

First picked from a shrub,
For white, green, or black tea
From China, it comes.

Tea – *Camellia sinensis*

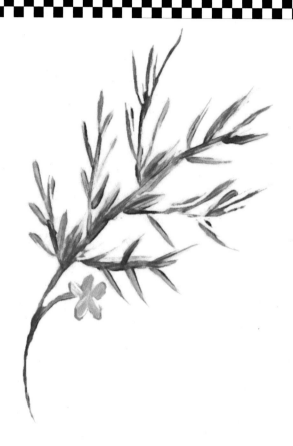

Tea tree – *Melaleuca alternifolia*

T is for Tea tree.

Dilute in base oil,
Use topical when
Fungal growth you must foil.

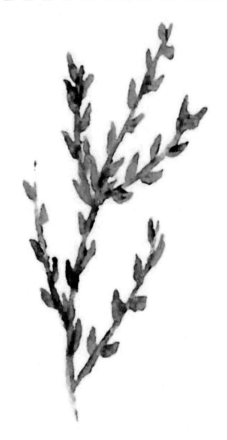

Thyme - *Thymus vulgaris*

T is for Thyme.

An herb to behold,
For most things heal with thyme
Says wisdom of old.

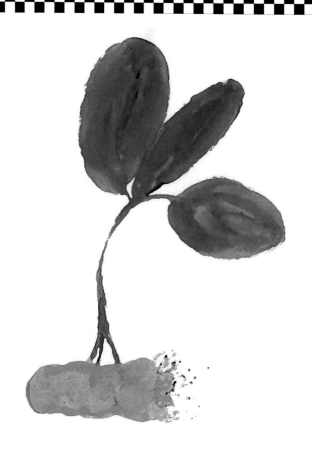

Turmeric – *Curcuma longa*

T is for Turmeric.

It stains a deep yellow
But indulgence today
May mean good health tomorrow.

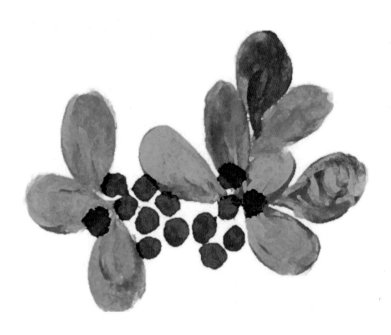

Uva Ursi - *Arctostaphylos uva-ursi*

U is for Uva Ursi.

Though not widely known,
The seeds are most useful
For dissolving soft stones.

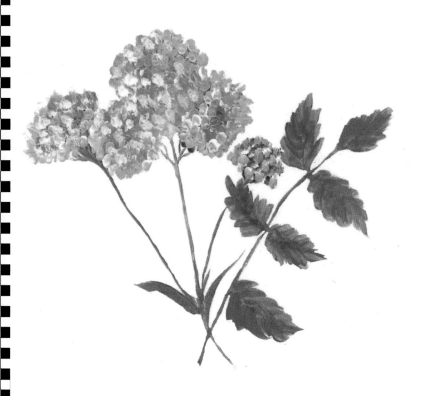

Valerian - *Valeriana officinalis*

V is for Valerian.

Best to know your intent,
Great for sleep or toothaches,
Never mind the strange scent.

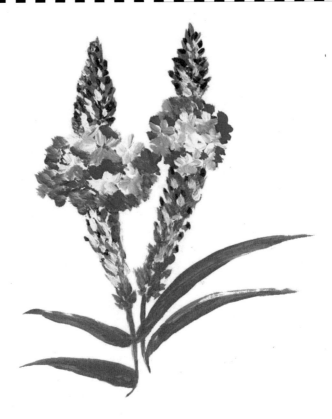

Vervain – *Verbena officinalis*

V is for Vervain.

It has a calming effect
With mint leaves and honey
Makes a tea, excellent.

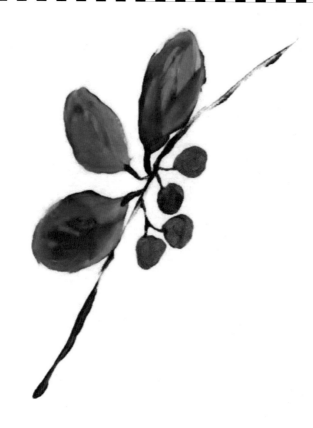

Wild Cherry Bark – *Prunus serotina*

W is for Wild Cherry.

A child's cough it does suit
Use the bark as the remedy
And flavor with the fruit.

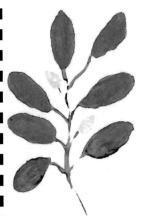

W is for Willow.

You may not have heard,
Bark eases aches and pain
To whom it may concern.

White Willow - *Salix alba*

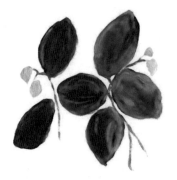

Wintergreen – *Gaultheria procumbens*

W is for Wintergreen.

Please don't go extreme,
To calm muscle tension
A small amount is all you need.

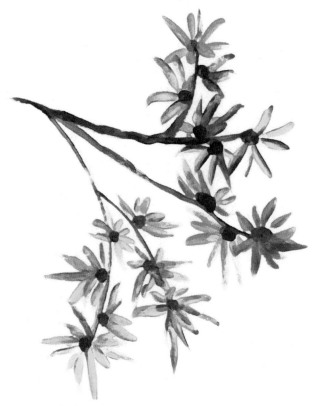

Witch hazel – *Hamamelis virginiana*

W is for Witch hazel.

Consider it for a minor bleed
And to reduce irritation,
This astringent does the deed.

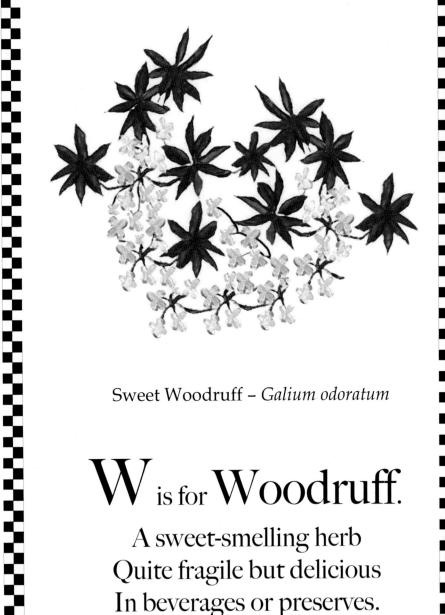

Sweet Woodruff – *Galium odoratum*

W is for Woodruff.

A sweet-smelling herb
Quite fragile but delicious
In beverages or preserves.

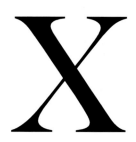

X

Stop for a moment!
Let X mark the spot,
Where you think of an herb
That was missed not forgot.

Here's a few...

Angelica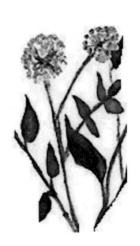

Comfrey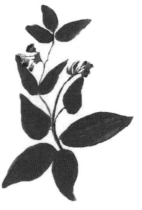

Horsetail

Cinnamon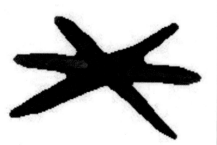

Feverfew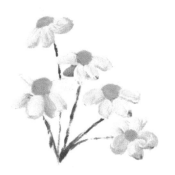

Lungwort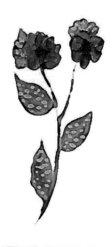

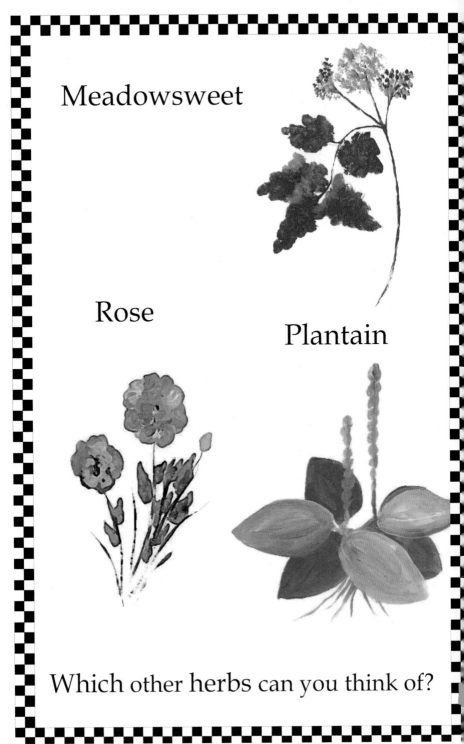

Meadowsweet

Rose

Plantain

Which other herbs can you think of?

Just a few pages left,
But it's easy to see
All that you can learn,
Now for herbs Y and Z.

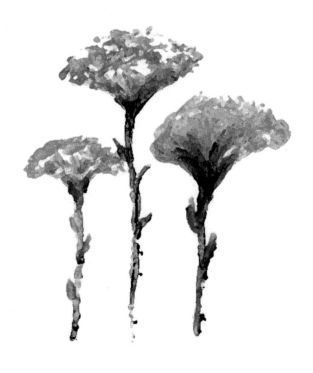

Yarrow - *Achillea millefolium*

Y is for Yarrow.

Use when wounded or sick,
Cured the heel of a god
In an ancient Greek myth.

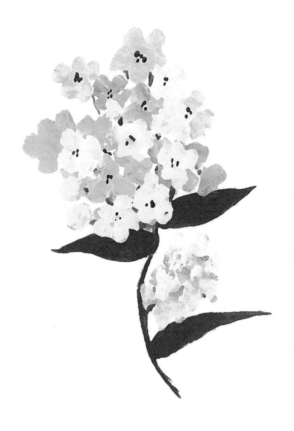

Yerba Santa – *Eriodyctyon californicum*

Y is for Yerba Santa.

Leaves are most sacred
In North and South America
For its cures and its fragrance.

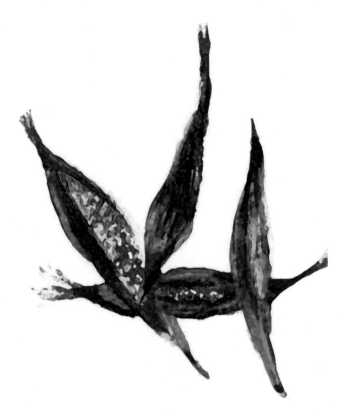

Corn silk - *Zea mays*

Z is for Zea mays.

Translated from Latin,
Means Corn silk! The tea,
Goes down smoothly, like satin!

Made in the USA
Coppell, TX
25 May 2023

17277488R00050